Self-Healing: Embrace the Power of Self-Healing through Meditation, Visualization, and Personal Empowerment

While every precaution has been taken in the preparation of this book, the publisher assumes no responsibility for errors or omissions, or for damages resulting from the use of the information contained herein.

SELF HEALING

First edition. October 19, 2023.

ISBN: 979-8224655496

Written by Gonzalo Estrada.

Table of Contents

To Moni, Ana and Gonz

Contents

Chapter 1: Understanding Self-Healing

Discover the fundamental principles of self-healing and how it can transform your life for the better.

In a fast-paced and often chaotic world, it's easy to forget that deep within each of us lies the incredible power of self-healing. This innate ability has been disregarded or even dismissed by many, overshadowed by the prominence of conventional medicine and external solutions. However, it's time for us to acknowledge and embrace the potential that lies within, to tap into our own healing capacity and transform our lives from the inside out.

Self-healing is not a new concept; ancient civilizations recognized and utilized its power. Yet, in our modern society, we have become disconnected from this innate ability, relying on external remedies and quick fixes instead. It is vital for us to reawaken our understanding of self-healing and reclaim our personal power to heal ourselves.

At its core, self-healing is the process by which we facilitate our own physical, emotional, and spiritual well-being. It involves harnessing the energy within us, activating our body's natural healing mechanisms, and restoring harmony to all aspects of our being. It's about recognizing that we are not helpless victims of circumstances, but active participants in our healing journey.

One of the key principles of self-healing lies in the power of the mind. Our thoughts and beliefs play a significant role in shaping our reality and influencing our health. By harnessing the potential of our mind through practices such as meditation and visualization, we tap into a realm where profound healing can occur. Meditation allows us to quiet the noise of the outside world and tune in to the wisdom within ourselves. It is in the silence of our minds that we find clarity, inner peace, and the ability to activate our body's healing response.

Visualization is another powerful tool in the realm of self-healing. By vividly imagining ourselves in a state of perfect health, we send powerful signals to our subconscious mind and align ourselves with the healing energy of the universe. Our thoughts become magnets, drawing in the positive energy necessary for healing and transformation. Through visualization, we can strengthen our connection with our body, understanding its needs, and nurturing it with love and compassion.

In addition to the power of the mind, self-healing requires personal empowerment. It demands that we take responsibility for our well-being and actively participate in our healing process. Empowerment means making conscious choices, adopting healthy habits, and surrounding ourselves with positivity. It means honoring our body's signals, listening to its whispers, and responding with love and care.

True self-healing is a holistic approach that encompasses not only our physical body but also our emotions and spirit. It recognizes that we are multidimensional beings, interconnected and in constant flux. When we address the root causes of our imbalances, whether they are physical, emotional, or spiritual, we create the space for true healing to occur.

As we delve deeper into the practice of self-healing, we discover that it is a journey of self-discovery, transformation, and personal growth. It is not a quick fix or a one-size-fits-all solution. It requires patience, dedication, and an open mind. But the rewards are immeasurable.

In the second half of this chapter, we will explore practical techniques, exercises, and case studies to deepen our understanding of self-healing. We will delve into the power of energy healing, the role of intuition in facilitating our healing journey, and the importance of self-compassion and self-love. By expanding our knowledge and implementing these practices into our lives, we can unlock the full potential of self-healing and experience profound transformation.

But for now, let us take a moment to acknowledge the incredible power that resides within each of us. The power to heal, to grow, and to embrace a life of vitality and well-being. Stay tuned for the next part of this chapter, where we will explore the practical aspects of self-healing and uncover the secrets that lie within.

Remember, the journey of self-healing begins with a single step—one that you are about to take. Embrace the power within, and prepare to embark on an extraordinary adventure of self-discovery and transformation. Now, as we continue our exploration of self-healing, let us delve into practical techniques, exercises, and case studies that will deepen our understanding and help us harness the power within.

Energy healing is a profound aspect of self-healing that taps into the universal life force energy that flows through all living beings. This energy, known as chi, prana, or ki, is the vital force that sustains our physical, emotional, and spiritual well-being. By working with energy healing modalities such as Reiki, acupuncture, or qigong, we can access and balance this energy within ourselves.

Through the gentle laying of hands or the use of specific points on the body, energy healing helps to remove blockages, release stagnant energy, and restore the natural flow of life force energy. It facilitates a state of deep relaxation, promoting healing on all levels and allowing us to reconnect with our innate capacity to heal.

Another powerful tool we possess in our self-healing journey is our intuition. Intuition is the inner knowing that arises beyond the realm of logic and reasoning. It is the voice of our higher self, guiding us towards what is truly beneficial and aligned with our well-being.

By developing and trusting our intuition, we can tap into valuable insights and make choices that support our healing process. Listening to our inner voice, quieting the doubts and fears of the rational mind, we open ourselves to the wisdom and guidance that resides within us.

Self-compassion and self-love are integral to the practice of self-healing. It is vital to cultivate a loving and nurturing relationship with ourselves, as this forms the foundation for our well-being. Treating ourselves with kindness, gentleness, and acceptance allows us to heal from past wounds, release self-judgment, and open up to the transformative power of self-love.

Practicing self-compassion means acknowledging our human imperfections, embracing our vulnerabilities, and offering ourselves forgiveness and understanding. By extending this compassion to ourselves, we create an environment of love and acceptance where healing can thrive.

Throughout our self-healing journey, it is essential to remember that healing is not linear or defined by set timelines. Each of us is unique, and our healing process unfolds at its own pace. Patience, compassion, and self-acceptance are crucial in navigating the ebbs and flows of healing.

As we incorporate these practices into our daily lives, we allow self-healing to become a way of living rather than a destination. It becomes a conscious choice to prioritize our well-being, to honor our bodies, minds, and spirits, and to pursue a life of vitality and wholeness.

In the grand tapestry of life, self-healing holds the power to transform not only ourselves but also the world around us. By embracing our innate healing capacity, we become beacons of light, radiating the energy of love, compassion, and well-being.

So, as we conclude this chapter on understanding self-healing, let us take a moment to honor the incredible journey we are embarking upon. Know that you possess the ability to heal, grow, and transform your life from within. Trust in the power that resides within you, and let it guide you towards a life of profound empowerment and well-being.

Remember, dear reader, you are not alone on this journey. There is a vast community of fellow seekers, healers, and lovers of life who are on this path alongside you. Find solace and support in connecting with others who share your passion for self-healing, whether it be through workshops, online forums, or local support groups.

Now, as you close this chapter, take a deep breath and allow the wisdom and insights you have gained to settle within. Reflect on the transformation that awaits you as you continue your journey towards self-healing.

In the chapters that follow, we will explore specific techniques, exercises, and resources that will empower you to deepen your practice of self-healing. We will delve into the power of breathwork, the benefits of plant medicine, and the healing properties of sound. Stay tuned for the next installment, where we will unlock the secrets that lie within, and continue on this extraordinary adventure of self-discovery and transformation.

Remember, my friend, you have the power within you to heal and thrive. Embrace it, nurture it, and watch as your life blossoms into a beautiful tapestry of well-being, joy, and vitality.

Chapter 2: The Power of Mind-Body Connection

Uncover the profound influence the mind has on the body and explore the interconnectedness between the two.

The human mind is a remarkable and powerful tool that shapes our experiences, beliefs, and perspectives. It has the ability to influence not only our thoughts and emotions but also our physical well-being. This intricate connection between the mind and body has long been recognized and studied, revealing the immense potential for healing and self-transformation.

When we talk about the mind-body connection, we acknowledge the undeniable impact our thoughts, attitudes, and emotions can have on our physical health. Countless studies have shown that chronic stress, negative thinking, and suppressed emotions can contribute to the development of various ailments, including cardiovascular diseases, immune system disorders, and even cancer.

On the other hand, studies have also discovered the incredible healing power that lies within our minds. Research on the placebo effect, for instance, demonstrates how the belief in a treatment or therapy can lead to actual physical improvements, even when the treatment itself has no medically active ingredients. This phenomenon highlights the extraordinary ability of our minds to influence the body's response to healing.

One of the most accessible and effective ways to harness the power of the mind-body connection is through the practice of meditation. Meditation allows us to calm the constant chatter of the mind, and in doing so, it brings us into a state of deep relaxation and inner peace. By focusing our attention on the present moment and cultivating a sense of mindfulness, meditation enables us to become more attuned to the signals our bodies are sending us.

Through meditation, we can tap into our body's wisdom and better understand the underlying causes of any physical discomfort or disease. As we quiet our minds and listen more attentively, we may discover that certain emotions, beliefs, or past traumas are manifesting as physical symptoms. This awareness provides us with the opportunity to address these underlying issues and initiate the healing process from within.

Alongside meditation, visualization is another powerful tool that can strengthen the mind-body connection. By vividly imagining positive outcomes and envisioning our bodies in a state of optimal health, we can stimulate healing at a deep subconscious level. Visualization allows us to activate our body's natural healing mechanisms and boosts our immune system's response, facilitating recovery and well-being.

Personal empowerment plays a significant role in the mind-body connection as well. When we recognize and embrace our ability to influence our own health and well-being, we begin to take responsibility for our own healing journey. Through personal empowerment, we shift from a passive role to an active participant in our own wellness.

Empowerment involves making conscious choices that support our physical and mental well-being, such as adopting healthy habits, nourishing our bodies with nutritious foods, engaging in regular exercise, and developing positive self-talk and affirmations. By actively engaging in self-care practices and adopting a proactive mindset, we can build resilience, enhance our overall well-being, and experience the transformative power of self-healing.

As we delve deeper into exploring the mind-body connection, we will uncover specific techniques and practices that can help us tap into this incredible potential for self-healing. From mindfulness exercises to positive affirmations, and from energy healing modalities to the power of gratitude, we will delve into the vast realm of possibilities that lie within our own minds and bodies.

In the second half of this chapter, we will explore how ancient wisdom and modern science converge to shed light on the mind's impact on the body. We will uncover the fascinating research that reveals the intricate ways in which our thoughts, emotions, and beliefs affect our physical health. Get ready to embark on a journey of self-discovery and empowerment as we uncover the significance of the mind-body connection and its tremendous potential for healing.

And with that, our exploration of the mind-body connection has only just begun...In the second half of this chapter, we will delve deeper into the fascinating research that reveals the intricate ways in which our thoughts, emotions, and beliefs affect our physical health. Prepare to embark on a journey of self-discovery and empowerment as we uncover the significance of the mind-body connection and its tremendous potential for healing.

Ancient wisdom and modern science align to shed light on the profound connection between our minds and bodies. Throughout history, various cultures have recognized the power of this connection and utilized practices such as meditation, visualization, and energy healing to promote well-being and healing.

As we explore the mind-body connection, we come across studies that highlight the impact of thoughts and emotions on our physical health. Negative emotions like anger, fear, and stress can contribute to the development of chronic diseases and weaken our immune system. On the other hand, cultivating positive emotions like love, joy, and gratitude can enhance our overall well-being and boost our immune response.

Further research has shown that our beliefs and perspectives play a crucial role in shaping our health. The placebo effect is a prime example of how our minds can influence our physical well-being. When individuals believe they are receiving a treatment or therapy, even if it is a sugar pill or a pretend treatment, their bodies often respond positively and experience actual improvements. This clearly demonstrates the power of our minds to influence healing and recovery.

In addition to the placebo effect, studies have also revealed the impact of our mindset on pain perception. Research conducted on patients with chronic pain has found that those who adopted a more positive and optimistic attitude experienced reduced pain levels and improved functionality. This astonishing discovery underscores the significance of our thoughts and attitudes in managing and even alleviating physical discomfort.

The mind-body connection is not just limited to our thoughts and emotions. It extends to how we perceive and interpret our experiences. Our beliefs about ourselves, the world, and the meaning we attach to the events in our lives can shape our physical health. For instance, individuals who believe they have control over their health and can actively participate in their healing journey often experience better outcomes.

As we continue to explore the mind-body connection, we come to realize that our bodies hold deep wisdom that can guide us towards healing. By cultivating a sense of mindfulness and a heightened awareness of our bodily sensations, we can tap into this wisdom and gain insights into the underlying causes of any physical discomfort or illness.

Through these insights, we may discover that certain emotional patterns, unresolved traumas, or limiting beliefs are being manifested as physical symptoms. This awareness empowers us to address these underlying issues and initiate the healing process from within. By combining our awareness with various self-healing techniques, we can create a harmonious balance between our minds and bodies, facilitating overall well-being and vitality.

Practices such as mindfulness meditation, positive affirmations, energy healing, and gratitude play a pivotal role in strengthening the mind-body connection. These practices help us cultivate a state of deep relaxation, release suppressed emotions, and foster a sense of inner peace.

By engaging in these techniques regularly, we actively contribute to our own healing and empower ourselves to take charge of our well-being.

In conclusion, the mind-body connection is a profound and intricate relationship that offers immense potential for healing and self-transformation. The evidence from both ancient wisdom and modern science clearly demonstrates how our thoughts, emotions, beliefs, and perspectives can influence our physical health.

By embracing the power of this connection and integrating practices like meditation, visualization, and personal empowerment into our lives, we can tap into the wellspring of healing that resides within us. Remember, you have the capacity to take charge of your own health and well-being. Embrace the power of your mind and inner wisdom, and embark on a journey of self-healing and transformation. The path to vibrant health and true empowerment starts from within.

Chapter 3: Cultivating a Meditation Practice

In today's fast-paced world, finding moments of inner calm and stillness may seem like a daunting task. However, it is precisely during these moments of pause and introspection that we can tap into our natural ability to heal from within. Meditation, a powerful tool that has been practiced for centuries, not only helps us find inner peace but also enhances the process of self-healing.

Learning and nurturing a meditation practice is a journey that begins with a single step, a conscious decision to take time for oneself and explore the depths of our own being. Whether you are completely new to meditation or have dabbled in it before, this chapter will provide you with practical techniques to help you start and maintain a consistent meditation practice. By incorporating meditation into your daily life, you can unlock the transformative power of self-healing and embark on a path of personal empowerment.

Before we delve into the techniques, it is essential to understand the purpose and benefits of meditation. At its core, meditation is a means to cultivate mental clarity, focus, and self-awareness. It allows us to observe our thoughts without judgment, creating a space for inner exploration and emotional well-being. Through regular practice, we can develop resilience, reduce stress, improve concentration, and tap into our innate healing abilities.

To embark on this journey, find a quiet and comfortable space where you can be free from distractions. It could be a dedicated meditation corner in your home, a peaceful outdoor spot, or even a quiet room in your workplace. The key is to choose a space where you feel safe and relaxed, allowing for a deeper sense of connection with yourself.

As you settle into your chosen space, begin by finding a comfortable sitting position. You can sit on a cushion or a chair, ensuring that your spine remains straight yet relaxed. Start by taking a few deep breaths, inhaling through your nose, and exhaling through your mouth. Allow the tension in your body to melt away with each breath, bringing yourself into the present moment.

Now, let's explore two fundamental meditation techniques that will serve as the foundation for your practice. The first technique is focused attention meditation, also known as mindfulness meditation. In this practice, you redirect your attention to a specific focal point, such as your breath or a chosen mantra.

As you focus on your breath, observe the inhalation and exhalation without trying to change its rhythm. Notice the sensations of the breath entering and leaving your body. If your mind wanders, gently guide your attention back to the breath, without judgment. Remember, the purpose is not to eliminate thoughts but rather to cultivate a compassionate awareness of the present moment.

The second technique we will explore is visualization meditation. Visualization is a powerful tool that allows you to create mental imagery and harness the mind-body connection. Begin by bringing to mind a specific image or scene that evokes feelings of peace and healing. It could be a serene beach, a lush forest, or even a gentle waterfall.

Immerse yourself in this visualized space, engaging your senses and noticing the intricate details. Feel the warmth of the sun on your skin, hear the soothing sounds of nature, and take in the vibrant colors of your surroundings. Allow yourself to be fully present in this created reality, soaking in the healing energies it provides.

As you cultivate and refine your meditation practice, remember that consistency is key. Set aside a few minutes each day, gradually increasing the duration as you become more comfortable. Just like any skill, meditation requires practice and patience. Be gentle with yourself and embrace the process, knowing that every moment spent in stillness brings you closer to self-healing and personal empowerment.

As we conclude the first half of this chapter, take a moment to acknowledge the progress you have already made. You have embarked on a powerful journey of self-discovery and healing through meditation. When you join us in the second half of this chapter, we will delve even deeper into advanced meditation techniques and explore how to incorporate visualization and personal empowerment into your practice. As you continue to cultivate your meditation practice, you will find that there is a wealth of techniques and approaches to explore. In the second half of this chapter, we will delve deeper into advanced meditation techniques and explore how to incorporate visualization and personal empowerment into your practice.

One powerful technique to enhance your meditation practice is loving-kindness meditation. This technique involves generating feelings of compassion and love towards yourself, others, and even the world as a whole. Begin by finding a comfortable position and taking a few deep breaths to center yourself. Then, bring to mind someone you care deeply about—a loved one, a close friend, or even a beloved pet. As you focus on this person, silently repeat phrases such as, "May you be happy, may you be healthy, may you live with ease."

Next, gradually expand your circle of loving-kindness to include yourself. Repeat these same phrases, directing them towards your own well-being and happiness. Acknowledge any resistance or self-critical thoughts that may arise and respond to them with gentleness and compassion. Remember, learning to love yourself unconditionally is a beautiful act of self-healing.

Once you feel comfortable generating feelings of loving-kindness towards yourself and your loved ones, you can extend this practice to include all beings. Imagine your love and compassion flowing outwards, encompassing everyone in the world. Silently repeat the phrases, "May all beings be happy, may all beings be healthy, may all beings live with ease." Allow this feeling of boundless love and kindness to permeate your being, knowing that you are contributing to the collective healing of all living beings.

Another technique that can deepen your meditation practice is the use of guided meditations. Guided meditations provide a structure and support as you explore different aspects of your being. You may choose to listen to pre-recorded guided meditations or use written scripts to create your own guided meditation practice.

To begin, find a guided meditation that resonates with you. It could focus on relaxation, healing, or personal empowerment. Set aside a dedicated time and space to listen to the guided meditation, making sure you won't be disturbed. As you listen, allow yourself to be fully present and open to the guidance offered. Follow the instructions, allowing the words and imagery to guide you deeper within.

Guided meditations can be a wonderful tool for exploring specific aspects of yourself and your healing journey. They can help you release limiting beliefs, tap into your inner wisdom, and connect with your innate power. Experiment with different guided meditations to find ones that resonate with you and support your self-healing intentions.

As you continue to refine your meditation practice, it is important to integrate the qualities of self-compassion and non-judgment. Be patient with yourself as you explore different techniques and experiences. Remember that there is no right or wrong way to meditate. The beauty of meditation lies in the process, not the outcome. Each moment spent in stillness is a moment of self-nurturing and growth.

Throughout your meditation practice, keep in mind that personal empowerment is both a catalyst and an outcome. As you cultivate a sense of inner knowing and connection, you will naturally feel more empowered in all aspects of your life. The stillness and clarity that meditation brings allow you to listen to your intuition, make conscious choices, and take inspired action.

In conclusion, your meditation practice is a sacred journey of self-discovery, healing, and personal empowerment. As you embrace the power of meditation, you unlock the potential to heal from within and create a life filled with joy, balance, and abundance. Remember, consistency and self-compassion are essential as you explore different techniques and approaches. Trust in your own ability to heal and know that you have everything you need within you.

Chapter 4: Harnessing the Art of Visualization

Visualization is a powerful tool that connects us to the deepest parts of our being, helping us unlock our inner potential and facilitating self-healing. Through the art of visualization, we tap into the immense power of our minds to create positive changes within ourselves and our lives.

Imagine for a moment closing your eyes and envisioning a serene tropical beach. You can feel the warm sand between your toes, hear the gentle lapping of waves against the shore, and taste the salty ocean breeze on your lips. As you delve deeper into this visualization, your body begins to relax, tension melting away, and a sense of peace washes over you. This is the transformative magic of visualization.

Visualization allows us to vividly picture our desires, dreams, and aspirations, creating a mental image that feels so real that our minds and bodies respond as if it were happening in the present moment. The mind becomes a canvas, and with focused intention, we paint a picture that becomes our reality.

Now, you might wonder how this can be possible. How can mere thoughts and mental images have such a profound impact on our well-being? The answer lies in the intricate connection between the mind and the body. Our thoughts shape our perception of the world and influence our emotions and physiological responses. Visualization harnesses this mind-body connection to promote healing and personal empowerment.

When we visualize ourselves in a state of perfect health and well-being, our brain releases a surge of neurotransmitters and hormones that support our physical and mental well-being. Studies have shown that visualization can positively impact our immune system, reduce stress levels, and even enhance our cognitive abilities.

Through visualization, we can connect with our innate ability to heal from within. By envisioning ourselves as healthy and whole, we activate our body's natural healing mechanisms, bringing about physical and emotional balance. Visualization acts as a catalyst for change, helping us transcend limiting beliefs and embrace a new reality.

To harness the art of visualization for self-healing, it is essential to create a sacred space where you can fully immerse yourself in the process. Find a quiet corner of your home or nature, free from distractions, and dedicate that space solely to your visualization practice. Consider adding elements that evoke a sense of tranquility, such as candles, essential oils, or soothing music.

Once you have found your sanctuary, sit in a comfortable position, relax your body, and take a few deep breaths. Allow any tension or stress to melt away, envisioning it leaving your body as you exhale. Now, close your eyes and begin to focus on the desired outcome of your visualization practice.

Be specific and detailed in your visualizations. Imagine yourself in perfect health, engaging in activities you love, and feeling vibrant and alive. Visualize every aspect of your desired outcome, including the sights, sounds, smells, and sensations associated with it. Engage all your senses in this visualization, making it as vivid and real as possible.

As you delve deeper into your visualization, notice any emotions that arise. Embrace and fully experience these emotions, allowing them to fuel your healing journey. Visualization is not just about picturing an outcome; it's about immersing yourself in the experience and feeling the transformative power within.

In this first half of our exploration into the art of visualization for self-healing, we have discovered the incredible potential it holds. By tapping into the power of our minds, we can actively participate in our healing process and cultivate a deep sense of personal empowerment.

Remember, this is only the beginning of your journey. The power of visualization knows no bounds, and in the second half of this chapter, we will delve deeper into specific techniques and practices to enhance the effectiveness of your visualizations. Prepare yourself for an immersive experience that will bring you closer to the power of self-healing.

Visualization Techniques for Enhanced Self-Healing

Now that you have established a sacred space and deeply immersed yourself in the power of visualization for self-healing, let us continue our exploration into specific techniques and practices that can enhance the effectiveness of your visualizations.

One powerful technique is the use of guided imagery. Guided imagery involves listening to or reading a script that leads you through a specific visualization experience. It provides a framework for your mind to follow, helping you dive deeper into your imagination and connect more fully with the healing potential within you. There are countless guided imagery resources available, ranging from pre-recorded audios to written scripts. Choose one that resonates with you and allows you to feel comfortable and secure in your visualization practice.

Another technique to enhance your visualizations is the integration of affirmations. Affirmations are positive statements that you repeat to yourself, reinforcing empowering beliefs and intentions. By incorporating affirmations into your visualizations, you infuse them with an added layer of intention and conviction. As you vividly imagine your desired outcome, use affirmations that align with that vision. For example, if you are visualizing perfect health, you might repeat affirmations such as, "I am strong, vibrant, and healthy in every way." As you engage your senses in the visualization, anchor these affirmations in your mind, allowing them to permeate every cell of your being.

Meditation can also be a powerful companion to visualization for self-healing. By quieting the mind and cultivating a state of inner stillness, meditation opens the door for deeper connection with your inner wisdom and intuition. Find a meditation practice that resonates with you, whether it be mindfulness meditation, loving-kindness meditation, or any other form that allows you to enter a state of presence and inner peace. Once you have settled into your meditation practice, transition seamlessly into your visualization, carrying the sense of calm and centeredness into your healing journey.

As you progress in your visualization practice, you may encounter moments of resistance or doubt. This is natural and part of the healing journey. When faced with such challenges, it is important to cultivate patience and self-compassion. Throughout your visualization, remind yourself that the process of healing unfolds in its own time and in its own way. Release the need for immediate results or perfect visualization, and trust in the innate intelligence of your body and mind. Embrace any emotions or thoughts that arise, understanding that they are part of the healing process and can provide valuable insights and opportunities for growth.

To deepen your connection with the art of visualization for self-healing, consider incorporating journaling into your practice. After each visualization session, take a few moments to reflect on your experience. Write down any insights, emotions, or sensations that arose during the practice. Journaling can help you gain clarity, provide a record of your progress, and serve as a source of inspiration and motivation during challenging times. It allows you to track your healing journey and celebrate the positive changes that emerge along the way.

In conclusion, the art of visualization is a profound tool for self-healing and personal empowerment. Through the power of your mind, you can activate your body's natural healing mechanisms and create positive changes in your physical and emotional well-being. As you continue to explore the limitless potential of visualization, remember to be patient, kind, and persistent with yourself. Trust in the process and embrace the transformative magic that lies within you.

The journey of self-healing through visualization is one of self-discovery, empowerment, and embracing your innate potential. By harnessing the art of visualization, you embark on a profound path of personal growth and transformation. So, continue to immerse yourself in the power of visualization for self-healing, knowing that you have the ability to create positive change from within. Embrace this journey wholeheartedly and allow the transformative magic of visualization to unlock the full potential that resides within you.

Remember, healing begins from within, and the power to heal lies in your hands. Harness it, embrace it, and embark on a journey of self-discovery like no other. Visualize, believe, and watch as your dreams become your reality. The power of self-healing through visualization awaits you.

Chapter 5: Tapping Into the Power of Affirmations

Positive affirmations have immense potential in the journey of self-healing. These simple yet profound statements can act as powerful catalysts to reprogram your subconscious mind, paving the way for optimal healing. Through the practice of affirmations, you can harness the transformative power of your thoughts and beliefs, setting the stage for profound personal empowerment.

Affirmations are more than mere words; they possess the ability to shape your reality. When you repeat affirmations consistently, their energy permeates your subconscious mind, challenging and transforming any negative or limiting beliefs that may hinder your healing process. By embracing the power of positive affirmations, you open the door to a realm of infinite possibilities.

One of the key aspects of utilizing affirmations for self-healing is the recognition that your thoughts have a direct influence on your overall well-being. Every thought you harbor generates a corresponding emotion, creating an energetic vibration that aligns with your inner state. When negative thoughts dominate your mind, they reverberate within, exacerbating pain, anxiety, and various other ailments. However, when you intentionally choose to focus on positive affirmations, you pave the way for healing and transformation.

Reprogramming your subconscious mind through affirmations begins with self-awareness. Observe the thoughts that arise within you and the beliefs you hold about your health and healing journey. Are these thoughts empowering and supportive? Or are they steeped in self-doubt, fear, and negativity? Acknowledging the patterns that arise is the first step towards transformation.

Once you have identified the thoughts and beliefs that no longer serve your healing process, you can consciously replace them with positive affirmations. Craft affirmations that are specific to your journey and resonate deeply with your desires for healing. For example, you might affirm, "I am healthy, vibrant, and completely in tune with my body's natural healing abilities."

The power of repetition cannot be underestimated when it comes to affirmations. Repetition helps solidify these empowering statements into your subconscious mind, gradually replacing old thought patterns with new ones. Incorporate affirmations into your daily routine, allowing them to become an integral part of your thoughts, words, and actions. Whether it's through silently repeating them during meditation, writing them in a journal, or placing sticky notes with affirmations around your living space, find a method that resonates with you.

Alongside repetition, visualization can enhance the effectiveness of affirmations. Visualize yourself embodying the state of healing you desire while affirming your intentions. See and feel the healing energy flowing through your body, picture yourself engaged in activities that bring you joy and vitality. Through the power of visualization, you align your mind, body, and spirit with the affirmations, amplifying their transformative force.

Remember, the journey of self-healing is unique to each individual. Thus, the affirmations you choose should reflect your personal experiences, desires, and goals. Tailor them to suit your needs and aspirations, crafting statements that empower you, uplift your spirit, and amplify your belief in your innate ability to heal from within.

As you continue to embrace the practice of positive affirmations, watch how they gradually influence your perception of your health and well-being. Notice the shifts taking place within you, both mentally and physically. With each affirmation, you reclaim your power and reaffirm your commitment to your healing journey.

Through the combined power of meditation, visualization, and affirmations, you have the key to unlock the profound potential of self-healing. In the second half of this chapter, we will explore advanced techniques to deepen your practice and tap into the limitless well of your personal empowerment. But for now, let the power of affirmations guide you towards healing from within, as you discover the strength and resilience that reside within your very core.

Harnessing the Power of Affirmations

Now that you have established the foundation for incorporating positive affirmations into your self-healing journey, it is time to explore advanced techniques that will further deepen your practice. By delving into these techniques, you will tap into the limitless well of your personal empowerment, unlocking even greater healing potential within yourself.

One of the most effective ways to enhance the power of affirmations is to infuse them with emotion. As you recite your affirmations, allow yourself to truly feel the emotions associated with the words. Feel the joy, the gratitude, and the sense of empowerment that arises within you as you affirm your intentions. Emotion acts as a catalyst, amplifying the energetic vibration of affirmations and strengthening their impact on your subconscious mind. When you infuse your affirmations with genuine emotion, you send a clear message to your mind and body, solidifying your belief in the healing process.

In addition to emotional infusions, you can also supercharge your affirmations by incorporating physical movement. Engaging your body in the affirmation process deepens the mind-body connection and reinforces the messages you are sending to your subconscious mind. Consider incorporating gentle movements or yoga poses while affirming your healing intentions. For instance, as you affirm, "I am vibrant and full of vitality," you can gracefully flow into a pose that embodies those qualities. By integrating physical movement with your affirmations, you create a powerful synergy between your mind, body, and spirit, further aligning them towards your healing goals.

Another advanced technique is to combine affirmations with guided imagery. Guided imagery involves creating vivid mental pictures that align with your affirmations. Close your eyes and visualize yourself in a tranquil, healing environment. See yourself surrounded by healing light, as it penetrates every cell of your being, rejuvenating and restoring your body to its optimal state of equilibrium. As you hold these visualizations in your mind, repeat your affirmations, allowing them to harmonize with the imagery. The combination of affirmations and guided imagery creates a potent cocktail of healing energy that resonates deep within your subconscious mind, further catalyzing the transformation process.

Furthermore, journaling can be a powerful tool to support your affirmation practice. Set aside time each day to write down your affirmations, allowing yourself to delve deeper into the energy and meaning behind each statement. Journaling allows you to explore any resistance or limiting beliefs that may arise as you work with your affirmations. By acknowledging and releasing these obstacles, you create space for new and empowering beliefs to take root. In your journal, you can also document any shifts, insights, or breakthroughs you experience along your healing journey. This not only provides a tangible record of your progress, but also serves as a source of encouragement and motivation during challenging times.

Lastly, it is important to be patient and persistent with your affirmation practice. Rome wasn't built in a day, and neither is deep healing. Commit to repeating your affirmations daily, nurturing your mind with positive thoughts and beliefs. Remember, the subconscious mind is like a fertile garden that requires consistent care and attention. Just as you wouldn't expect flowers to bloom overnight, trust that with time and dedication, your affirmations will blossom into tangible healing results.

As you embark on this empowering journey of self-healing through affirmations, embrace the infinite possibilities that lie within you. Trust in your ability to reprogram your subconscious mind, paving the way for optimal healing and transformation. Each day, as you tap into the power of affirmations, you are reclaiming your power and reaffirming your commitment to your well-being.

Continue to tune in to the whispers of your soul, as it guides you towards the path of healing and personal empowerment. Remember, you are the author of your own story, capable of creating a life filled with health, abundance, and joy. With each affirmation you utter, you are awakening the dormant power within, stepping into your innate ability to heal from within.

In the next chapters, we will delve deeper into other transformational practices that will further support your self-healing journey. But for now, let the power of affirmations work its magic in your life. Embrace them as the sacred key that unlocks the door to unparalleled levels of self-healing and personal growth. Trust in the process, have faith in yourself, and always remember that you are an embodiment of divine resilience and infinite potential.

Chapter 6: Nurturing Self-Love and Compassion

In our journey of healing from within, it is crucial to embrace the practice of self-love and compassion. These qualities are like the fertile soil that allows the seeds of self-healing to take root and flourish. Just as a flower needs nurturing care and attention to blossom, so too do we need to cultivate and foster an environment of love and compassion within ourselves.

Self-love is often misunderstood as being selfish or narcissistic. However, true self-love goes beyond egoistic desires and delves into a deep appreciation and acceptance of oneself. It is about recognizing our inherent worth and treating ourselves with kindness, respect, and care. When we cultivate self-love, we develop a strong foundation for healing, as we believe in our own ability to grow, transform, and overcome any challenges that come our way.

Compassion is an essential companion to self-love. It is the act of extending kindness, empathy, and understanding towards ourselves and others. When we embrace compassion, we acknowledge the interconnectedness of all beings and recognize that suffering is a shared human experience. By showing compassion to ourselves, we create a nurturing environment that fosters healing and growth. Compassion allows us to be gentle and patient with our own struggles, offering ourselves the same compassion we would offer a dear friend.

So how do we nurture and cultivate self-love and compassion within ourselves? One powerful tool is the practice of meditation. This ancient practice allows us to quiet the mind, become more present, and develop a greater sense of self-awareness. Through meditation, we can tap into our deepest selves, discovering our own truths, desires, and needs. It is in this quiet space that we can truly listen to and connect with ourselves.

Incorporating visualization into our practice can deepen our connection to self-love and compassion. Visualization is a powerful tool that allows us to imagine and picture ourselves in a state of healing, love, and contentment. Visualizing ourselves surrounded by a warm, glowing light of compassion and self-acceptance enables us to embody these qualities more fully. It provides us with a blueprint for how we can show up for ourselves and others with love and kindness.

Alongside meditation and visualization, personal empowerment plays a significant role in nurturing self-love and compassion. Personal empowerment involves taking responsibility for our own well-being, growth, and happiness. It means recognizing our strengths, setting healthy boundaries, and making choices aligned with our values and desires. When we empower ourselves, we embody the love and compassion we deserve. We become active participants in our own healing, knowing that we hold the power to create positive change in our lives.

By embracing the practice of self-love and compassion, we lay the foundation for self-healing to flourish. Through meditation, visualization, and personal empowerment, we create a nurturing environment within ourselves. In this safe and loving space, we can explore our wounds, release past traumas, and cultivate a sense of self-worth. As we continue on this journey of healing, we invite you to open your heart and mind to the transformative power of self-love and compassion.

In the practice of nurturing self-love and compassion, it is important to actively cultivate these qualities in our daily lives. It is not enough to simply understand their importance; we must actively engage in practices that promote their growth and development.

One powerful way to nurture self-love and compassion is through the practice of self-care. Taking care of ourselves physically, emotionally, and mentally is a powerful act of love and compassion. This can involve simple activities such as nourishing our bodies with nutritious food, getting enough sleep, and engaging in regular exercise. It can also involve engaging in activities that bring us joy and help us relax, such as reading, practicing hobbies, or spending time in nature. By prioritizing self-care, we send a clear message to ourselves that we are deserving of love and care.

Another powerful tool in nurturing self-love and compassion is the practice of positive self-talk. The way we speak to ourselves has a profound impact on our self-perception and overall well-being. By intentionally replacing negative self-talk with positive affirmations and kind words, we can shift our internal dialogue towards a more loving and compassionate mindset. Treat yourself as you would a dear friend - with kindness, encouragement, and support.

Mindfulness is another practice that can deeply nourish self-love and compassion. By bringing our attention to the present moment without judgment, we cultivate a deeper sense of self-awareness and self-acceptance. Mindfulness allows us to observe our thoughts and emotions without attachment or criticism, fostering a compassionate understanding of ourselves. Through regular mindfulness practice, we develop the ability to respond to ourselves with empathy and kindness, even in times of difficulty.

In addition to these practices, cultivating gratitude can greatly enhance our ability to love and have compassion for ourselves. Taking time each day to reflect on the blessings in our lives, both big and small, helps shift our focus towards abundance and appreciation. This practice reminds us of the many reasons we have to love and be compassionate towards ourselves and others. Gratitude opens our hearts to the beauty and joy that exists within and around us.

It is also vital to surround ourselves with a supportive and loving community. Connecting with like-minded individuals who share similar values and aspirations creates an environment that fosters self-love and compassion. These individuals can offer guidance, understanding, and a safe space for us to express ourselves authentically. By cultivating relationships based on love and compassion, we continue to grow and expand our capacity for self-love.

As we nurture self-love and compassion within ourselves, it is important to remember that this journey is not linear. There will be setbacks and moments of resistance, but we can approach these challenges with the same love and compassion we cultivate towards ourselves. Remember that healing and growth take time, and it is okay to be gentle with ourselves along the way.

By prioritizing self-love and compassion, engaging in self-care, practicing positive self-talk, cultivating mindfulness, expressing gratitude, and surrounding ourselves with a supportive community, we create a nourishing environment for self-healing to flourish. Let us continue on this journey of self-discovery and healing with open hearts and minds, embracing the transformative power of self-love and compassion.

Chapter 7: Overcoming Inner Resistance

Identify and overcome the internal barriers that hinder your path to self-healing, empowering you to break through resistance.

In our journey toward self-healing, we often encounter moments of inner resistance that threaten to hold us back. These barriers manifest in various forms, stemming from deep-rooted fears, limiting beliefs, and past traumas. Yet, it is through acknowledging and understanding these obstacles that we gain the power to overcome them.

Within each of us lies the key to unlocking our true potential for self-healing. The first step is to recognize the presence of resistance within ourselves. It may take the form of self-doubt, fear of change, or even a lack of belief in our own abilities. Whatever shape it assumes, resistance acts as a formidable force, causing us to question our worthiness of healing, and ultimately inhibiting our progress.

To overcome and conquer this resistance, we must start by delving into its roots. Reflect upon the moments in your life when you felt hesitant or resistant to change. Was it a past failure that left you feeling unworthy of success? Or perhaps a fear of stepping into the unknown? Identifying these barriers provides a roadmap to understanding ourselves on a deeper level.

Once these barriers are identified, it is important to approach them with compassion and self-acceptance. We must recognize that these barriers were not created to hinder us but rather as protective mechanisms. Our natural inclination as humans is to avoid pain and discomfort. It is through this lens that we can begin to view our resistance as a well-intentioned effort to shield ourselves from potential harm.

With this understanding, we can begin the process of dismantling these barriers. Cultivating a consistent meditation practice serves as a powerful tool in this journey. Through meditation, we can create a safe space to observe our thoughts, emotions, and patterns of resistance without judgment. By developing this awareness, we are better equipped to challenge the validity and necessity of these barriers.

Visualization is another potent technique that aids in overcoming inner resistance. Take a moment to envision yourself free from the chains of resistance. See yourself fully immersed in the healing process, embracing your inner power, and breaking through the barriers that hold you back. As you visualize this transformation, allow yourself to feel the emotions of liberation and empowerment. Visualizing the desired outcome connects us with the inherent strength within, encouraging us to take tangible steps towards our goals.

Personal empowerment plays a crucial role in overcoming inner resistance. Taking ownership of our healing journey requires a mindset shift – one where we acknowledge our ability to actively participate in our own growth and transformation. Embrace the belief that you possess the strength and resilience to break through any barrier that stands in your way.

It is important to remember that overcoming resistance is not an overnight process. It requires patience, perseverance, and a deep commitment to self. We may face setbacks along the way, but it is in these moments that we must summon our courage and remind ourselves of the resilience within.

As we conclude this first half of our exploration into overcoming inner resistance, remember that healing from within is a transformative and ongoing journey. Embrace the power of self-reflection, meditation, visualization, and personal empowerment to confront the barriers that hinder your path to self-healing. By understanding and dismantling these barriers, you unleash the full potential of your inner strength. It is through this process of overcoming resistance that you will discover the true essence of healing from within.

With each step we take in the direction of self-healing, we become more attuned to the inner landscapes of our being. We have already explored the roots of our resistance and discovered the power of meditation, visualization, and personal empowerment in breaking through these barriers. Now, it is time to delve deeper into the transformative process of overcoming inner resistance.

One of the most potent tools we have at our disposal is self-affirmation. Through affirmations, we can rewrite the narratives that have held us back, replacing them with empowering beliefs that propel us forward. Take a moment to reflect on the negative self-talk that often accompanies moments of resistance. Perhaps you find yourself saying, "I am not strong enough," or "I don't deserve to heal." These are the seeds of self-doubt that hinder our progress.

Now, flip those statements on their head and craft affirmations that counteract the resistance. Repeat them to yourself daily, with conviction and belief. "I am strong and capable of healing." "I am deserving of love, joy, and wellness." These affirmations act as gentle reminders of our inherent worthiness and potential for growth. They break down the walls of resistance, brick by brick, until we are left standing in the open expanse of self-empowerment.

The journey of healing from within is often not a solitary one. Surrounding ourselves with a support system can greatly aid in overcoming resistance. Seek out individuals who uplift and understand you, creating a safe space for vulnerability and growth. Share your struggles and triumphs with them, draw inspiration from their journeys, and offer support in return. Together, you can navigate the hurdles of resistance and foster a sense of collective empowerment.

Additionally, seeking professional guidance can provide valuable insights and tools for overcoming inner resistance. A therapist, coach, or mentor can help you explore the deeper layers of your resistance and guide you through the process of dismantling these barriers. They offer unbiased perspectives and strategies to facilitate your self-healing journey.

As we strive to overcome resistance, it is essential to approach ourselves with kindness and patience. Healing is not a linear path, and setbacks are inevitable. It is in these moments that we must tap into us well of resilience and tap into self-compassion. Remind yourself that growth is a journey, and each stumble is an opportunity to learn and realign with your true self. Be gentle with yourself during this process, celebrating your progress no matter how small it may seem.

In conclusion, the process of overcoming inner resistance is a transformative and courageous endeavor. It requires us to face our deepest fears and challenge the beliefs that hold us back. Through self-reflection, meditation, visualization, personal empowerment, affirmations, and support, we can dismantle these barriers one by one, liberating ourselves from the constraints that hinder our self-healing.

Remember, you are not alone in this journey. Countless others have walked this path before you, and countless more will follow. Embrace your uniqueness, your power, and your worth. Believe in your ability to break through resistance and embrace the fullness of your healing potential.

As we reach the end of our exploration into overcoming inner resistance, take a moment to honor the progress you have made thus far. Celebrate your courage, your resilience, and your unwavering commitment to self-healing. Each step you take brings you closer to the radiant wholeness that awaits within you.

Now, my dear reader, armed with the knowledge and tools to overcome your inner resistance, go forth fearlessly on your path of healing. Embrace the transformation that awaits you, and let the power of self-healing illuminate every corner of your being. You are capable, you are deserving, and you are ready to embrace a life of wellness, joy, and empowerment.

Chapter 8: Healing through Forgiveness

Forgiveness is a profound and transformative power that holds the key to our self-healing journey. It is a crucial step in releasing emotional burdens, freeing ourselves from past hurts, and embracing a life of immense joy and fulfillment. When we are able to extend forgiveness, not only to others but also to ourselves, we open the door to immense healing and personal growth.

Within each one of us lies a capacity for forgiveness, a divine ability to let go of resentment, anger, and pain. However, it is important to acknowledge that forgiveness is not synonymous with condoning or forgetting the actions that have caused us harm. Instead, it is a conscious decision to release the grip these past experiences have on our hearts and minds. It is an act of reclaiming our power and stepping into a place of emotional freedom.

The journey towards forgiveness begins with a deep understanding of its transformative potential. Holding onto grudges and grievances only perpetuates our own suffering. It becomes a heavy burden that weighs us down and prevents us from fully embracing the beauty and joy that life has to offer. Choosing forgiveness does not mean we invalidate our pain or deny the impact of past events. Rather, it is an act of self-compassion, allowing ourselves the opportunity to heal and grow beyond our pain.

One of the profound ways forgiveness enables self-healing is by liberating us from the shackles of resentment. When we hold onto anger and resentment, we bind ourselves to an endless cycle of negativity. In this state, we are entrapped in our own suffering, unable to move forward and experience true healing. By letting go of resentment, we break these chains, paving the way for personal growth, love, and happiness.

Another powerful aspect of forgiveness is the ability to cultivate empathy and compassion towards others. Often, the person who has hurt us is also carrying their own burdens, their own wounds that led them down the path of inflicting pain upon others. By recognizing these shared human struggles, we shift our perspective and foster a sense of understanding. We acknowledge that hurt people hurt others, and we can choose to break this cycle through forgiveness and compassion.

In addition to forgiving others, it is equally essential to extend forgiveness to ourselves. We are all flawed beings, prone to making mistakes and experiencing regret. Holding onto self-blame and shame only hinders our self-healing journey. By practicing self-forgiveness, we offer ourselves the opportunity for growth, self-love, and acceptance. We recognize that we are deserving of compassion, just like anyone else.

As we embark on the path of forgiveness, it is important to remember that it is not always an easy journey. It takes courage, patience, and a willingness to confront and process our emotional pain. There may be moments of resistance or doubt, but perseverance is key. We must remind ourselves of the immense power and freedom that forgiveness provides, motivating us to continue on this transformative path.

We will delve deeper into the process of forgiveness, guiding you through the steps that will enable you to release emotional burdens and experience profound healing. Stay tuned, for the journey has only just begun, and the power of forgiveness awaits you.

In the second half of this chapter, we will explore practical strategies and exercises to help you cultivate forgiveness in your life. These techniques are designed to empower you to release emotional burdens and experience profound healing. Remember, forgiveness is a gift you give to yourself, and it is within your reach to access this liberating power.

One effective strategy for cultivating forgiveness is through the practice of mindfulness. Mindfulness allows us to fully experience and acknowledge our emotions without judgment or attachment. By cultivating a sense of presence and awareness, we can gently observe our feelings of anger, resentment, or pain without getting caught up in them. This practice creates a space for acceptance and compassion to arise, fostering a fertile ground for forgiveness to take root.

A practical exercise you can engage in is journaling. Writing down your thoughts and emotions can provide clarity and give you a fresh perspective. Begin by reflecting on the person or situation that has caused you pain. Write freely and honestly—express every emotion, every thought that arises without any judgment. Use this space to vent, release, and process your feelings.

Once you have poured out your emotions onto the pages, take a step back and read what you have written. Notice any recurring patterns or themes, and try to identify any underlying beliefs or expectations that may be contributing to your pain. Ask yourself if holding onto these feelings serves your highest good or if it is hindering your growth and well-being.

Now, imagine yourself sitting face to face with the person who has caused you harm. This may initially feel uncomfortable or even impossible, but remember that forgiveness is a journey, and this exercise is one step towards healing. Holding this image in your mind, express your forgiveness to them. Speak your words of forgiveness out loud or silently, trusting that the energy of forgiveness is reaching its intended recipient.

In addition to these reflective exercises, it is crucial to actively practice self-compassion. Too often, we are our own harshest critics, replaying past mistakes and blaming ourselves for the pain we have experienced. But healing cannot truly occur without self-forgiveness.

Take a moment now to send love and compassion to yourself. Recognize that you are human, and like everyone else, you are prone to making mistakes. Appreciate the lessons learned from these experiences and acknowledge your growth. Embrace the truth that you deserve forgiveness, understanding, and unconditional love. Imagine yourself wrapping your arms around your inner wounded self, offering comfort and reassurance.

As you continue your journey toward forgiveness, keep in mind that it is not a linear process. There may be setbacks, times when old wounds resurface, and moments of doubt. Do not be discouraged; instead, embrace these moments as opportunities for deeper healing and growth. Remember that forgiveness is not a one-time event but a continuous practice of letting go and creating space for love and joy to flow in.

In conclusion, forgiveness is a profound act of self-compassion and empowerment. It holds the power to liberate us from emotional burdens, free us from the cycle of negativity, and open the door to immense healing and personal growth. Through mindfulness, journaling, and self-compassion, we can cultivate forgiveness in our lives, allowing ourselves to fully embrace the beauty, joy, and fulfillment that life has to offer.

As you embark on your journey towards forgiveness, hold onto the belief that you have the inner strength and resilience to navigate this transformative path. With each step, you are reclaiming your power, healing your wounds, and tapping into the infinite well of compassion within you. The power of forgiveness awaits you; embrace it fully, for it is the key to your self-healing and inner liberation.

Chapter 9: Embracing Personal Empowerment

Within each one of us resides an incredible power, the power to heal ourselves from within. It is through personal empowerment that we can tap into this innate potential and take charge of our own healing journey. When we embrace personal empowerment, we connect with our true selves, unlocking a wealth of strength, resilience, and inner wisdom.

In today's fast-paced world, it is easy to feel overwhelmed and disconnected from ourselves. We often find ourselves seeking external solutions to our problems, believing that someone or something else holds the key to our healing. But the truth is, the power to heal lies within us. It is a force that, when embraced, can transform our lives in profound ways.

Personal empowerment begins with recognizing and acknowledging our own worth. We are inherently deserving of love, happiness, and well-being. By nurturing this self-worth, we create a solid foundation for personal growth and healing. It is essential to understand that we have the power to shape our own experiences and determine our own destinies.

One powerful tool that can guide us on our path towards personal empowerment is meditation. Through the practice of meditation, we learn to quiet the noise of the outside world and turn our attention inward. It is in this space of stillness that we can connect with our intuition and gain clarity about our desires, needs, and aspirations.

During meditation, we allow ourselves to let go of the stresses and worries that burden us. We become observers of our thoughts and emotions, without judgment. Through this practice, we cultivate self-awareness and develop the ability to respond to life's challenges with calmness and clarity. In turn, this empowers us to make choices that align with our true selves and promote our well-being.

Visualization is another powerful tool that can support our journey towards personal empowerment. By using our imagination, we can create vivid mental images of the life we desire. Visualizing ourselves as healthy, vibrant, and in harmony allows us to embody these qualities on a deeper level. It helps us manifest our intentions and strengthens our belief in our own ability to heal.

When we embrace personal empowerment, we begin to take ownership of our healing journey. It is no longer about relying solely on external remedies or waiting for someone else to save us. It's about reclaiming our power and actively participating in our own well-being. We become proactive in seeking out the support, resources, and practices that resonate with us and contribute to our growth and healing.

As we tap into our true potential through personal empowerment, we discover that healing is not a destination but a continuous, ever-evolving process. It requires patience, self-compassion, and a willingness to embrace change. We learn to embrace our vulnerabilities and acknowledge that they are part of our shared human experience. In doing so, we cultivate a greater sense of empathy and compassion towards ourselves and others.

Embracing personal empowerment is about recognizing that we have the capacity to create our reality. We are not victims of circumstance but creators of our own stories. As we step into our power, we inspire others to do the same, creating a ripple effect of healing and positive transformation in the world.

... As we journey further into the realm of personal empowerment, we discover the immense power of self-belief and the impact it has on our healing process. Believing in ourselves is not always an easy task, especially when faced with challenges and setbacks. However, it is through these challenges that we learn and grow the most.

When we choose to believe in our own abilities, we open ourselves up to endless possibilities. We release the limitations and doubts that hold us back and embrace a mindset of resilience and determination. By acknowledging that we have the strength and capability to overcome obstacles, we propel ourselves forward on the path of healing.

In order to strengthen our self-belief, it is important to surround ourselves with supportive and positive influences. This may include seeking out like-minded individuals who are on a similar journey of self-empowerment. Connecting with others who share our goals and aspirations can provide encouragement, inspiration, and a sense of community.

Moreover, it is vital to cultivate an inner dialogue of self-compassion and self-encouragement. We must be our own cheerleader, celebrating our achievements no matter how small they may seem. By acknowledging our progress and acknowledging our efforts, we nourish the seed of self-belief within us, helping it to flourish.

In addition to self-belief, self-acceptance is a crucial aspect of personal empowerment. Embracing all parts of ourselves, including our flaws and imperfections, allows us to cultivate a deep sense of self-love and compassion. When we accept ourselves fully, we detach ourselves from the need for external validation and find solace in our own approval.

Practicing self-acceptance requires us to let go of self-judgment and comparisons to others. Each of us is on a unique journey, and our experiences and growth cannot be measured against anyone else's. By focusing on our own progress and experiences, we are able to fully embrace and appreciate our individuality.

As we continue on our healing journey, it is important to remember that personal empowerment is not a linear process. There will be moments of doubt and moments of triumph. It is in these moments that we learn the most about ourselves and our capabilities. We must allow ourselves to stumble, to learn, and to grow from these experiences.

During these times, it is essential to practice self-care and self-nurturing. This may involve engaging in activities that bring us joy and peace, such as spending time in nature, practicing self-care rituals, or engaging in creative pursuits. By prioritizing self-care, we honor our own needs and ensure that our energies are replenished, allowing us to continue on our path towards personal empowerment.

In conclusion, embracing personal empowerment is a transformative journey that leads us to tap into our true potential and take charge of our healing. Through self-belief, self-acceptance, and self-care, we unlock an unparalleled source of strength within ourselves. As we continue to embrace our personal power, we inspire those around us and create a ripple effect of healing, resilience, and positive change in our lives and in the world.

Remember, you possess the innate ability to heal from within. Embrace personal empowerment and unleash your true potential. You are deserving of love, happiness, and well-being. Trust in yourself, and the journey of self-healing will unfold before you, one powerful step at a time.

Chapter 10: Creating a Sustainable Self-Healing Lifestyle

Life is full of ups and downs, challenges and triumphs. It's easy to get caught up in the chaos and forget about taking care of ourselves. However, adopting a sustainable self-healing lifestyle can have a profound impact on our well-being, allowing us to navigate life's journey with grace and resilience. In this chapter, we will explore practical strategies to integrate self-healing practices into your everyday life, fostering long-term well-being.

As you embark on this transformative journey, remember that self-healing is not a one-time fix; it's a continuous process of growth and self-discovery. To create a sustainable self-healing lifestyle, it is essential to cultivate a mindset of self-compassion and make intentional and consistent choices that prioritize your well-being.

One powerful tool to incorporate into your daily routine is meditation. Meditation provides a space for deep relaxation and allows you to connect with your inner self. Find a quiet spot where you can sit comfortably, close your eyes, and focus on your breath. As thoughts arise, gently acknowledge them and let them go. With regular practice, meditation can help reduce stress, enhance clarity of mind, and promote emotional balance.

Visualization is another effective technique to harness the power of your mind for self-healing. By creating vivid mental images of your desired outcomes, you can activate the innate healing potential within you. Take a few moments each day to imagine yourself in a state of perfect health, radiating with vitality and joy. Visualize the healing energy flowing through your body, restoring balance and harmony. Trust in the power of visualization to manifest positive changes in your physical, emotional, and spiritual well-being.

In addition to meditation and visualization, personal empowerment plays a critical role in creating a sustainable self-healing lifestyle. Empowerment involves taking responsibility for your own well-being and actively participating in your healing journey. One way to cultivate empowerment is by setting clear and achievable goals. These goals act as guiding beacons, providing direction and motivation towards your desired state of well-being. Break your goals down into smaller, actionable steps, and celebrate each milestone along the way.

It's important to remember that self-healing is not a solitary endeavor. Creating a supportive network of like-minded individuals can amplify the power of your healing journey. Seek out communities or support groups that align with your values and aspirations. Surrounding yourself with people who share similar goals and struggles can provide encouragement, understanding, and accountability. Together, you can inspire each other and strengthen the collective energy for positive change.

As you navigate the path of self-healing, don't forget the importance of self-care. Self-care goes beyond pampering or indulgence; it is a fundamental practice that nourishes your mind, body, and soul. Prioritize activities that bring you joy, whether it's taking a leisurely walk-in nature, practicing yoga, or indulging in a favorite hobby. Remember that self-care is not selfish; it replenishes your energy and equips you to better support and uplift others.

In the first half of this chapter, we have explored practical strategies to integrate self-healing practices into your everyday life. From the power of meditation and visualization to personal empowerment and the significance of self-care, these tools lay the foundation for a sustainable self-healing lifestyle. By embracing these practices, you embark on a transformative journey towards long-term well-being.

Now, take a moment to reflect on what resonated with you in this first half of the chapter. Consider how you can begin implementing these strategies in your life starting today. When you embrace the power of self-healing and commit to nurturing your mind, body, and soul, you unlock a boundless potential for growth, joy, and resilience. The second half of this chapter holds even more insights and wisdom to support you on your path. Stay tuned, as the next part will delve deeper into practical techniques and mindset shifts for transformative self-healing. In the second half of this chapter, we will delve deeper into practical techniques and mindset shifts that will further support and empower you on your transformative self-healing journey. By embodying these strategies, you will continue to cultivate a sustainable self-healing lifestyle, fostering long-term well-being and resilience.

One essential practice to incorporate into your daily routine is the art of gratitude. Gratitude has the power to shift your perspective, allowing you to focus on the positive aspects of your life and fostering a sense of contentment and fulfillment. Take a few moments each day to reflect on the things you are grateful for, whether it's the support of loved ones, the beauty of nature, or the simple joys that brighten your days. By acknowledging and appreciating these blessings, you invite more positivity and abundance into your life.

Embracing a growth mindset is another crucial aspect of self-healing. A growth mindset involves believing in your ability to learn, grow, and overcome challenges. Instead of viewing setbacks and obstacles as failures, see them as opportunities for growth and self-discovery. Cultivate self-compassion and be gentle with yourself during times of struggle. Remember that each experience is a valuable lesson that propels you forward on your path to healing and personal evolution.

Finding your purpose and aligning your actions with your values can greatly contribute to your overall well-being. Take some time to reflect on what truly matters to you and what brings you a sense of meaning and fulfillment. Once you have a clear understanding of your purpose, make intentional choices that align with your values. By living authentically and in alignment with your true self, you will find a deep sense of fulfillment and purpose in your daily life.

As you continue your self-healing journey, it is important to prioritize self-compassion and embrace the concept of self-forgiveness. We all make mistakes and face challenges along the way, but harboring guilt or holding onto past resentments only hinders our healing process. Practice forgiveness towards yourself and others, letting go of any emotional baggage that no longer serves you. By releasing these burdens, your free up space within yourself to welcome healing, joy, and love.

In addition to these personal practices, it is essential to create a physical environment that supports your self-healing journey. Surround yourself with items, colors, and scents that bring you peace and uplift your mood. Declutter your physical space and create a sanctuary where you can relax and recharge. Consider incorporating elements of nature, such as plants or natural materials, to bring a sense of harmony and grounding into your surroundings.

Finally, embrace the concept of self-acceptance. Accepting yourself fully, with all your imperfections and strengths, allows for deep healing and growth. Let go of societal expectations and self-imposed limitations, and instead, celebrate your uniqueness and individuality. When you accept yourself as you are, you create an environment of love and self-compassion, inviting healing and transformation in every aspect of your life.

As we come to the end of this chapter, I encourage you to take a moment to reflect on the strategies and practices that resonated with you the most. Consider how you can begin implementing them into your life, starting today. Remember that self-healing is a continuous journey, and by embracing these practical techniques and mindset shifts, you will foster a sustainable self-healing lifestyle that nourishes your mind, body, and soul.

The power to heal lies within you, and with each intentional step you take, you unlock greater potential for growth, joy, and resilience. Embrace the journey, trust in your innate ability to heal, and know that you are supported every step of the way. Continue nourishing yourself with self-compassion, gratitude, growth, purpose, forgiveness, and self-acceptance, and watch as your self-healing journey unfolds into a beautiful tapestry of well-being and wholeness.

Stay tuned for the next part of your journey, where we will dive even deeper into the transformative power of self-healing. Until then, may you walk this path with courage, grace, and an unwavering belief in your own capacity to heal from within.

Disclaimer

Don't miss out!

Visit the website below and you can sign up to receive emails whenever Gonzalo Estrada publishes a new book. There's no charge and no obligation.

https://books2read.com/r/B-A-OZBBB-PWPPC

BOOKS 2 READ

Connecting independent readers to independent writers.

Did you love *Self Healing*? Then you should read *Analiza Resuelve Ejecuta*[1] by Gonzalo Estrada!

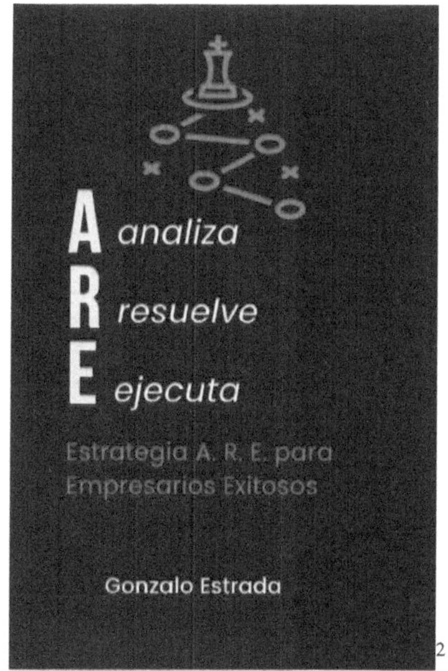

[2]

Descubre el poder transformador de la Estrategia A. R. E. (Análisis, Resolución del Problema y Ejecución) y desata todo tu potencial como emprendedor. En este libro, Gonzalo Estrada te lleva de la mano a través de un viaje fascinante hacia el éxito empresarial y la construcción de un patrimonio sólido. Con 19 capítulos repletos de consejos prácticos, ejemplos inspiradores y herramientas probadas, aprenderás a dominar cada etapa crucial del proceso empresarial.

Desde la importancia del análisis y la identificación de oportunidades hasta la creatividad en la resolución de problemas y la planificación meticulosa de la ejecución, cada capítulo te acerca más a convertirte en un verdadero generador de ingresos y a alcanzar tus metas

---

1. https://books2read.com/u/m0aGOM

2. https://books2read.com/u/m0aGOM

financieras. Aprenderás a superar el miedo al fracaso, a tomar acción de manera inmediata, a seguir un plan de seguimiento y ajuste, y a mantener una persistencia y consistencia que te llevarán a nuevos niveles de éxito.

Además, descubrirás la importancia de la automatización y escalabilidad, la delegación efectiva de tareas, la administración del tiempo y la mentalidad emprendedora que marcan la diferencia entre un negocio promedio y uno excepcional. Con ejemplos reales de casos hipotéticos y aplicaciones prácticas en diferentes áreas, este libro es una guía completa para aquellos que desean salir adelante de sus deudas, formar un patrimonio y triunfar en el mundo de los negocios.

Si estás listo para transformar tu mentalidad empresarial, dejar atrás las limitaciones y alcanzar el éxito que siempre has deseado, ¡entonces este libro es para ti! Empieza hoy mismo tu viaje hacia el éxito con la Estrategia A. R. E. y conviértete en el empresario que siempre has soñado ser.

Also by Gonzalo Estrada

Self Healing
Visualiza tu Éxito
Cultivando Líderes
Afirmaciones y Empoderamiento
Semillas de Cambio
Cómo convertir TikTok en una máquina de hacer dinero
Cómo hacer dinero con Pinterest
Cómo hacer un ensayo
Cómo Pedir un Aumento de Sueldo
Currículo Poderoso
Entrenamiento sin Violencia
Entrevista Laboral
Gana Dinero con X (Twitter)
Ganar Masa Muscular
Volver a Empezar; el arte de reinventarse
Analiza Resuelve Ejecuta
Aromatherapy, The natural path to your pet´s well being
Holistic Feeding
The ABC of Educating Your Pet
The Art of Cosmic Connection
The Art of Feng Shui applied to your Pets
From Scarcity to Abundance
The English Bulldog in The Family
The French Bulldog
Therapeutic Massages for Pets

About the Author

Gonzalo Estrada is a prolific and renowned author, whose books cover topics that resonate with humanity. With a prominent presence in both physical and online media, Estrada has made a significant mark in contemporary literature. His works, of great significance on platforms such as Amazon, Barnes & Noble, and many others, reflect his deep knowledge and passion for the subjects he tackles. From the transformative power of gratitude to the unique personality of the French Bulldog, Estrada has proven to be a versatile and captivating writer who has connected with readers from all over the world.